End

Hair Loss

Stop and reverse hair loss naturally

Nazeem Nour

Disclaimer

Although in this book you will only find natural and risk free advices and suggestions, the author of this book is not responsible for any incident that might happen after following the steps. If you suffer from any condition or if you have doubts, please consult a practitioner before following the steps of the program

My story

Few years ago, in my mid-twenties i started losing my hair, it was very stressful and i wasn't feeling well. I felt like i was losing a part of myself. My confidence got hit very hard.
Each time i looked at my hair in the mirror, i felt sad almost depressed. And when i found hair on my pillow it also made me sad. I was asking myself? Why is this happening, why?
I 'm sure that you are experiencing the same thing as me and you understand what i am talking about.
But i was motivated; i had the willingness to do anything to find a solution. And i knew deep down that i will find the solution and that i will stop losing my hair and even reverse hair loss. Thankfully i had the resources. After many years of research not only on hair loss but health in general, I finally found the solution that i am about to reveal to you in this book.
I can't describe to you this sensation when you know that you will never lose your hair again and

when you see it regrow. You feel happy, you feel reborn.

I remember the day i went to the barber after two years of cutting my hair alone at home (i cut it completely). It was strange: I felt like all the work that i have been doing to stop my hair loss and to make my hair regrow faster finally paid You need to know that hair is like a plant, it needs some nutriments (food; oxygen; sleep) but also it doesn't like other things like pollution, stress bad nutrition.

In this book i will show you exactly what you need to do in order to prevent, to stop and reverse hair loss

So let's start

Here is all you need to know to stop and reverse hair loss

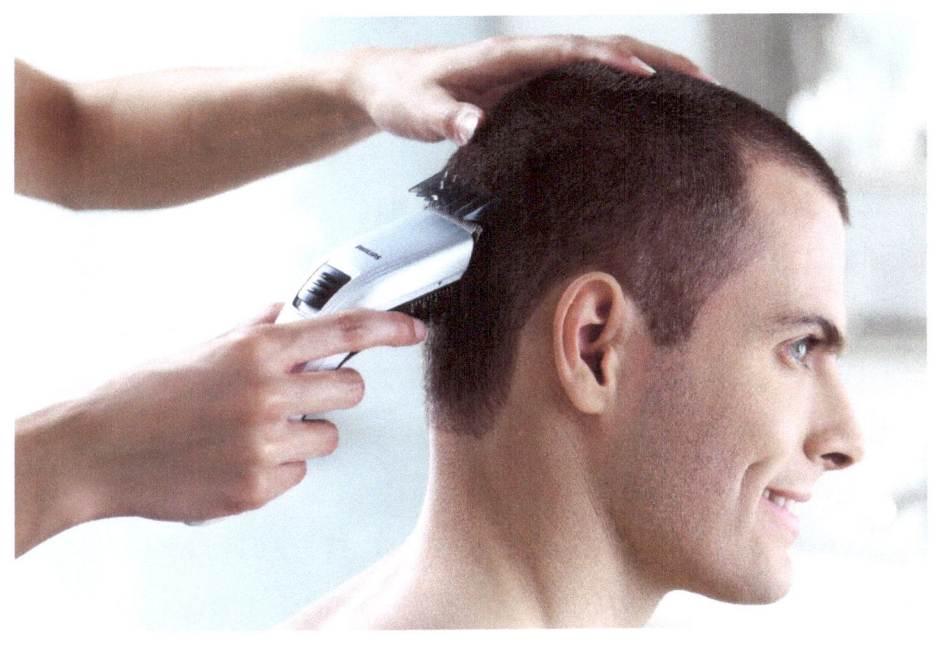

1

Cut your hair

When you feel that you start losing your hair, cut it. Cut it to a minimum, if you can cut it all then do it. Why?

Cutting your hair will prevent you from losing more hair immediately. I know it's the solution that you want or that you don't want to cut your hair but it only temporary. Not only it will stop your hair loss but it strength it.

I know that in some cultures it is advised to cut your hair completely, because it's good for the head and the hair.

You might have also noticed that each time you cut your hair, your hair feels stronger and look nicer.

So have some courage and don't hesitate to cut as much as you can. When you cut it all and you feel embarrassed or something, you can always wear a hat...

You can hear some people that say hats make you lose your hair. It can be true. And the reason is because the heat that is in your hat make you sweat, the sweat makes your hair wet and the hair fall easily when it's wet. But when you cut all your hair you don't lose hair. Also when the weather is cold your hair stay dry and you lose nothing.

This is only temporary. Once you stop your hair loss you can let your hair grow again

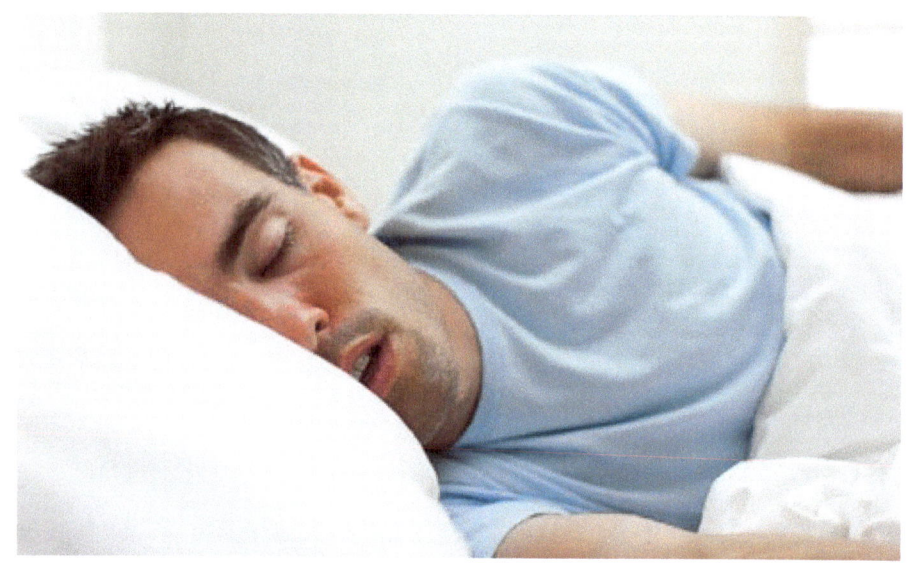

2

Sleep

Sleep a lot: sleeping is good for the hair and it will help you manage stress better (stress causes hair loss). The best thing to do is to not set the alarm, sleep until you wake up alone. You will easily notice that when you don't sleep well your hair (and your skin) doesn't look good and falls easily.

So make sure to go to sleep early this way you can get at least eight hours of sleep and more. Don't miss this step very important.

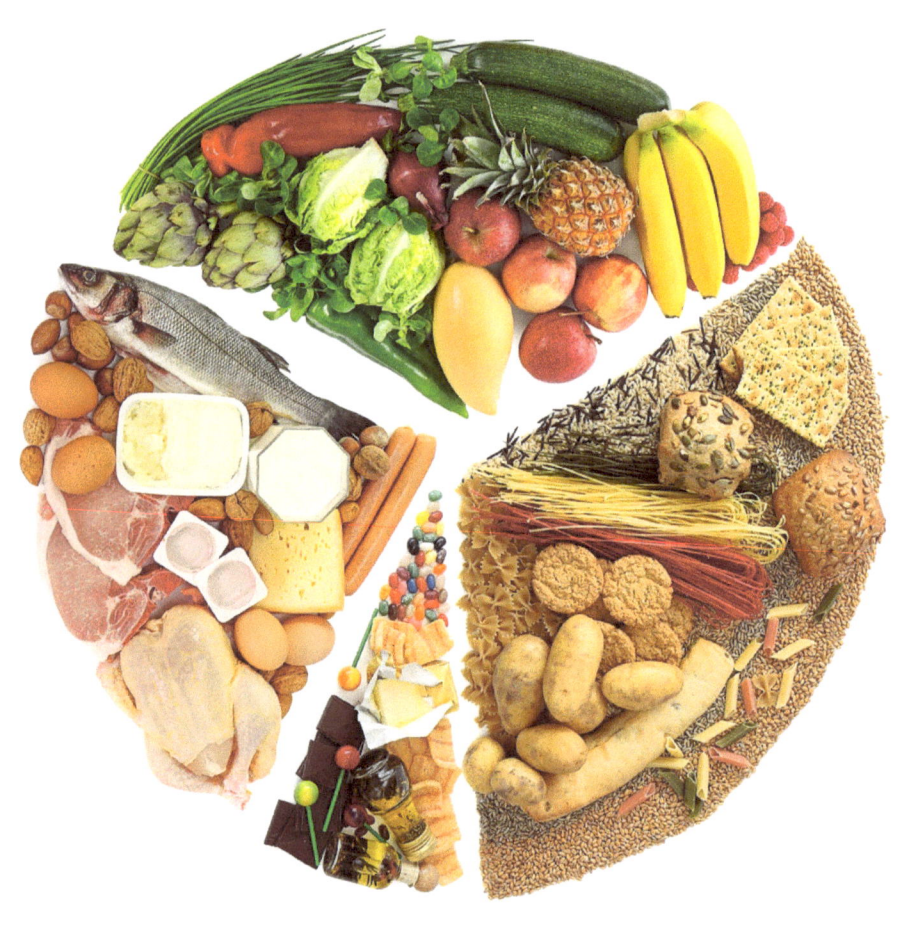

3

Food

Food is very important in fighting hair loss. You need to take this part very seriously. Here what will make a difference and will stop your hair loss:

_ Good quality food: seek food that is rich in nutrients like organic food or food without too much chemicals. The vitamins and minerals that are in your food will nourish your hair therefore stop and reverse hair loss. Seek also fresh food or food of the season which contain more nutrients. Try also to eat raw food more often!

_ Protein: they are essentials to your hair and nails whether it's chicken, meat or fish. I recommend animal protein because i noticed that it's better than vegetal protein (tofu, beans, seitan, eggs ...). Go for a good portion

with each meal: between 100g up to 300g.
_Cereals: cereals are also key to stopping and reversing hair loss. Go for brown rice and wheat. Don't eat too much wheat or anything that is based on wheat like pasta, bread because it can make you fat. If you don't want to get fat go for the rice

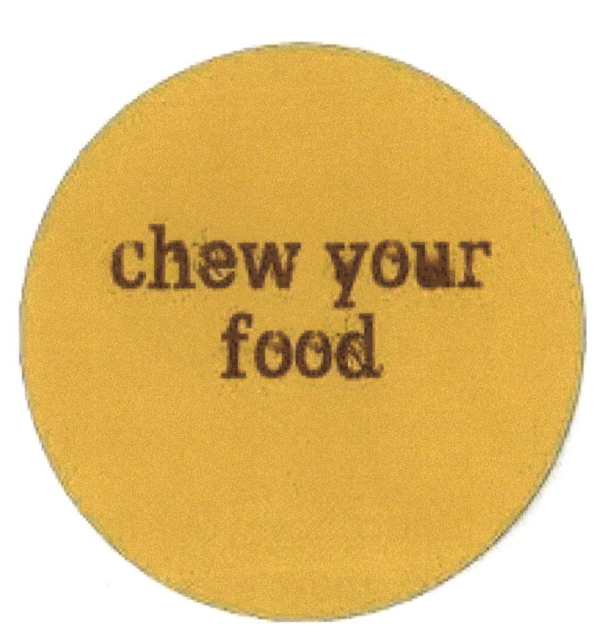

4

Chew

Chew your food: Chew your food hard, this will strengthen the muscle around your teeth and then your head, your hair in the same time. Food is becoming softer and softer (like junk food) seek good food that you can chew hard. When you are chewing your food, hold your teeth clunged together for three to five second, this will reinforce the muscles in your head, therefore your hair.

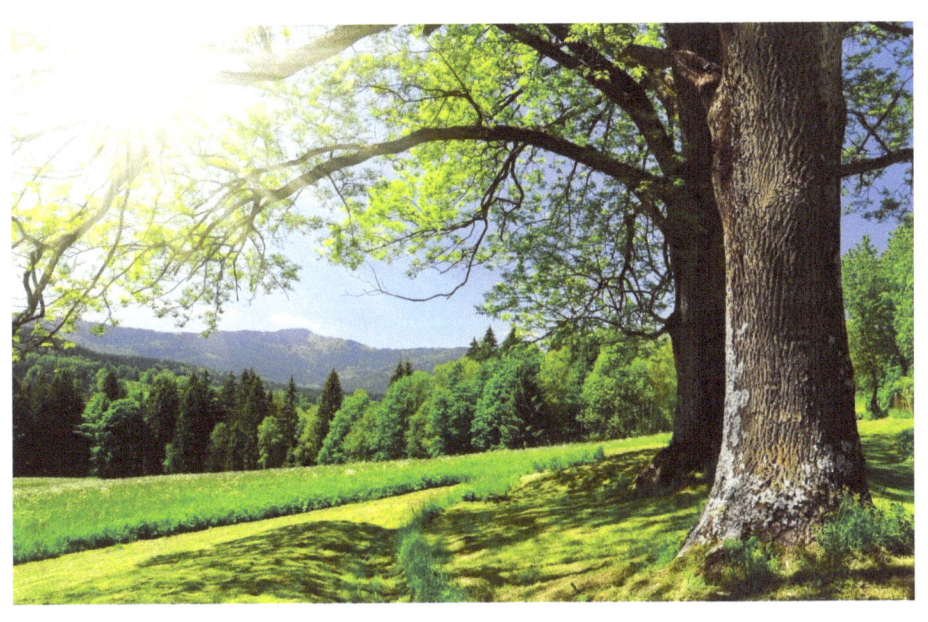

5

Fresh air

Seek fresh air: pollution is not good for hair. Avoid big cities if you can't, go to parks, forest... Do this at least 5 days a week for minimum 20 min. the more the better. Good quality air is very important for your hair. Sadly today the air is polluted, combine to that bad food and stress, there you have a recipe for disaster and for hair loss. Try to spend your holidays in the countryside or on the mountain. You should spend at least one month in a natural environment. Two months is good .Do breathing exercises, any breathing exercise you like.

One exercise that i like in particular: Breathe in from one nostril and hold it as much as you can then breathe out from the other nostril. Do it in the other sens: breathe in from the other nostril (you just exhaled from) hold then breathe out from the other side.

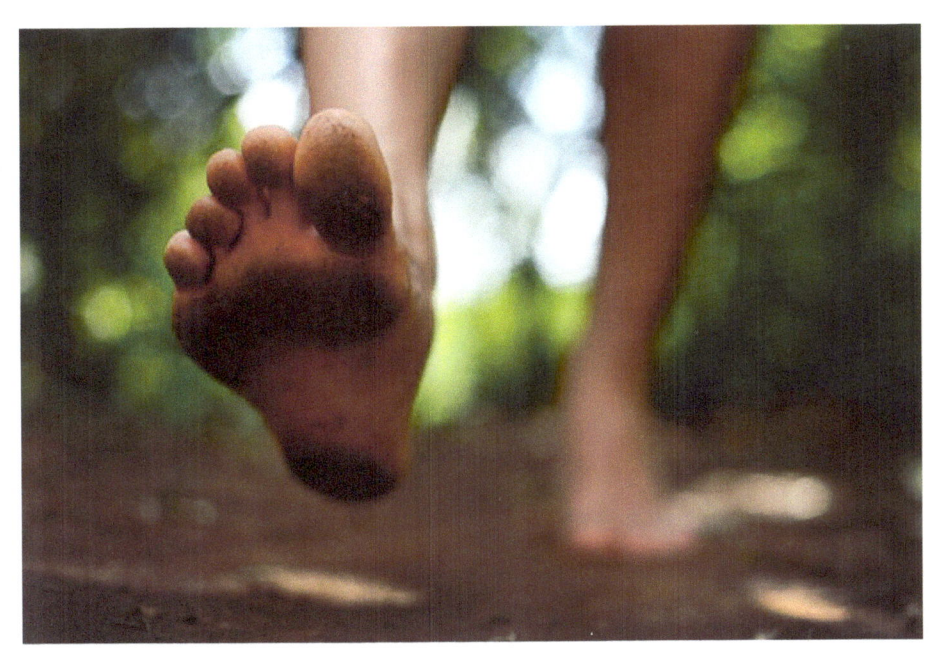

6

Ground yourself

Earthing: take off your shoes and ground yourself to the earth, it's good for your hair. Do this at least 5 days a week for 20 min. the more the better. Earthing is a new and a natural way to energize your body and your hair. you will find a lot of information on earthing and it's benefits, if you have never heard of it , i advice you to do some research on it , this way you will have a better idea on what i am talking about .

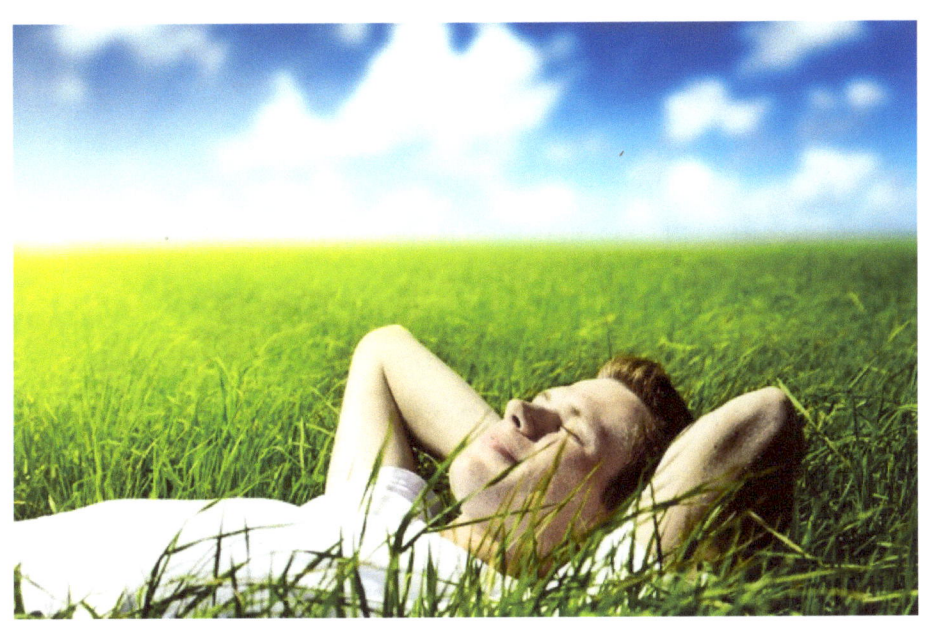

7

Rest

Rest: learn to rest during the day. Take a nap or a hot bath... Take breaks to avoid stress. Resting is important and it allows you to conserve physical energy.

I personally noticed that i lost less hair on my days off than on my working days. So if you care about your hair, conserve your energy. You might need to think of a way to work less and earn more, there are many solutions out there that will show you how to do it. Check out the book of Tim Ferriss *"The Four Hour Workweek"* for a start.

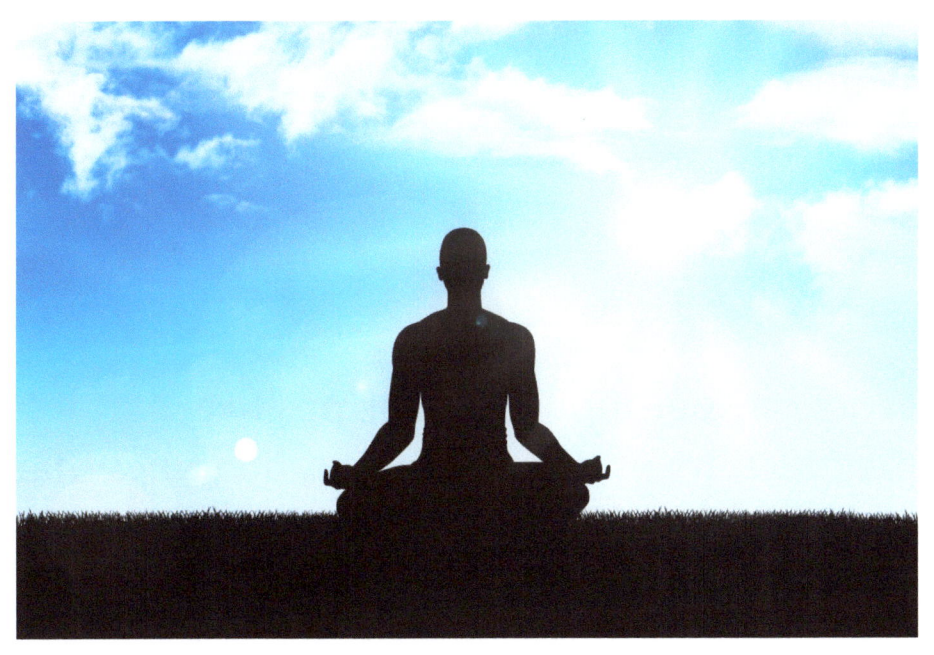

8

Stop worrying

Work on your thought, think positive, meditate, focus on the present, do things that make you feel good, listen to relaxing music.... Worrying stresses you and makes you lose hair.

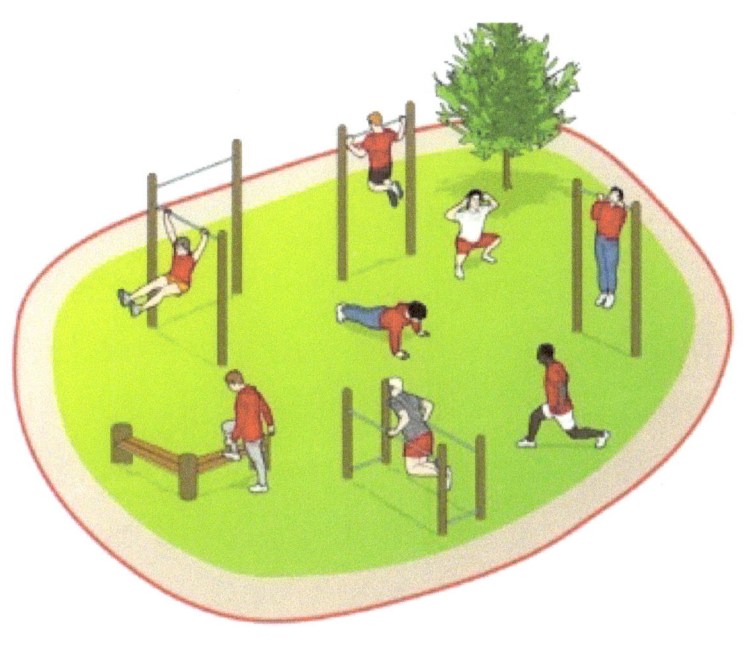

9

Exercise

Combine cardio with lifting/strength. Exercises like push-ups, burpees, mountain climber ... are good for hair loss. The swing of the kettlebell is also good. If you go to the gym focus on three exercises: dead lift, bench press and squat with this three exercises you work out your body and you increase blood circulation in your head and scalp.

The goal is to perform some type of vigorous activity for a minimum of 15 to 30 minutes, three to five times a week. This vigorous activity should be executed between 60% to 80% of your Maximum Heart Rate **(MHR)**
How to calculate your **MHR**:

a) - subtract your current age from 220. This number is your MHR.
b) - Multiply this number by 0.60. This is 60 percent of your MHR.
C) - take the number you came up with in step a). Multiply it by 0.80. This is 80 percent of

your MHR.

These numbers of 60 percent and 80 percent represent the range of your Target Heart Rate (THR). (An important note: many high blood pressure medications work by lowering the heart rate, which would mean that your MHR and target rates may need to be lowered as well. If you are taking any blood pressure medications, contact your physician to find out how best to adjust these numbers.)

When engaging in exercise, you will need to keep track of your heart rate to make sure you are staying within the 60 percent to 80 percent THR range. This is commonly done by lightly pressing the index finger of the right hand over the artery just under the skin on the skin on the inside of the left wrist. The rate is easily determined by counting the beats for 15 seconds, the multiplying that number by 4. This will be your heart rate. (Or count the beats for one minute)

If you don't like this way of counting your heart beats, there is an alternative rule of thumb: if you can hold a conversation, you aren't working hard enough. If you can sing, you are not working hard enough either. If you are out of breath, or have to stop and catch your breath, you're definitely working too hard. Stay in between!

Also it's important that you find an activity that you enjoy. There are a lot of activities out there, so find something that you enjoy. The main point here is to get your circulation going.

Exercise outside for maximum oxygen intake which will stimulate your scalp. But don't forget that chewing your food hard is the best exercise for hair loss.

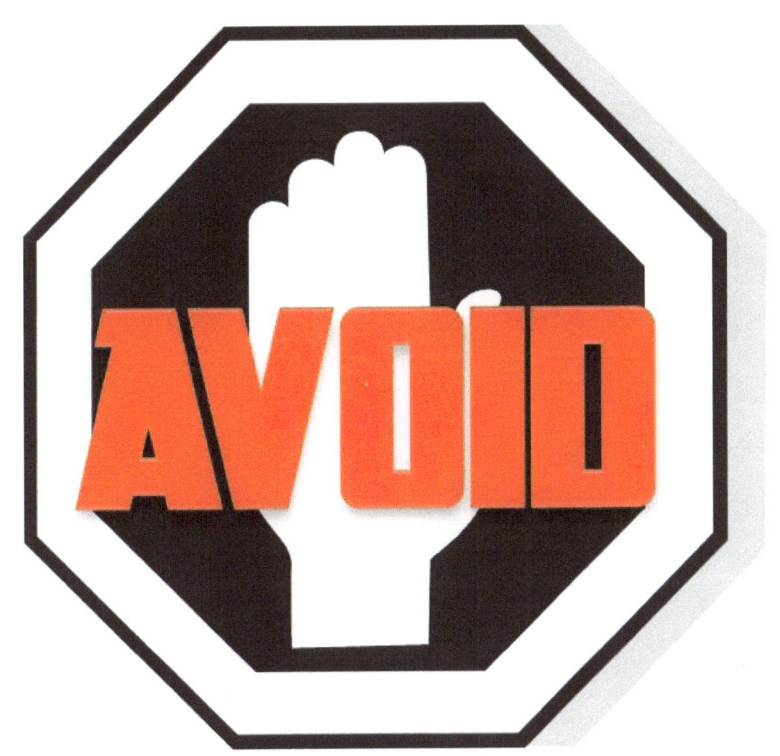

10

Avoid

What to avoid: Sugar, coffee, TV and sex

_ Sugar: Brian Tracy calls it a poison. Sugar is not only bad for your body and your health but it is also bad for your hair. The less you eat it the better.

_ Coffee: For the sake of your hair choose tea over coffee

_TV: too much TV could promote hair loss. Especially if you watch action movie or anything that could increase your stress level.

_ Sex: you could lose your hair when you have too much sex. How do you know if you are having too much sex? Well it's hard to know because it depends on many facts. But if you are suffering from hair loss, try to reduce your ejaculations. Reduce it by half or more. For example if you are having sex 4 times a week cut it to two times a week or one time a week . It might be difficult but it's just temporary. When you feel that you don't suffer from hair loss you can resume your regular sexual activity.

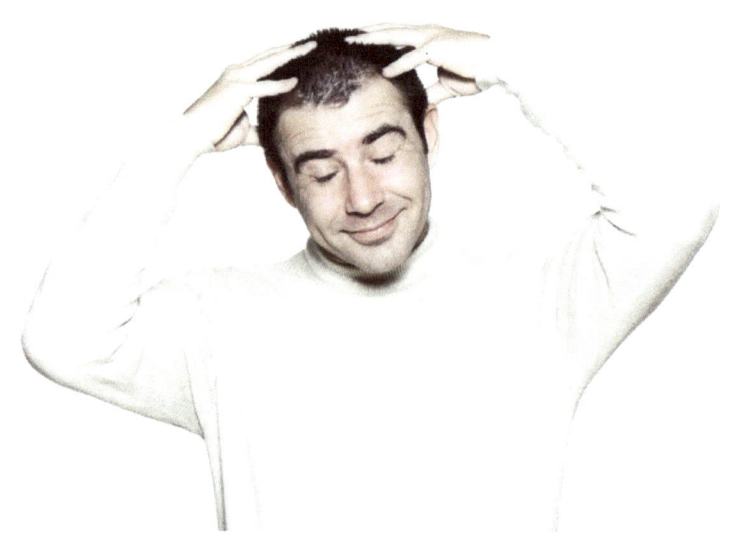

11

Massage

Massage your scalp: massaging will bring more blood to your scalp and stop hair loss. There are many exercises out there you can do any massaging exercise you want. The most important rule to follow is: don't use your nails when massaging. Your nails might hurt your hair.

Here are some exercises:

_ Hanging: Lie on your back on a bed or table hang your head off the edge so that blood circulation is increased through the neck and scalp. Breathe deeply and relax. Lie there for several minutes

_ Forehead Manipulation: Hold your left hand across the back of your head to steady your neck relaxes your head into your hand. Place your right hand across your forehead, stretching your thumb and forefinger across your brow line. Move your hand slowly and firmly upward to one inch past your hairline. Repeat four or five times.

_ Scalp manipulation: Place the palms of your hands firmly against your scalp above each ear. «Lift" the scalp in a circular movement, first with the hands at the side of your head, then with one hand at the top front and the other at the center back, right at the nape of your neck.

_Hairline Circles: Beginning at the hairline, place this fingers of both hands on the center of your hair line - right at your forehead. Massage around the hairline, concentrating on the areas of hair loss as you work your fingertips in a gentle circular motion. Work all the way around your hairline, including the temples, behind your ears, across the back of your neck.

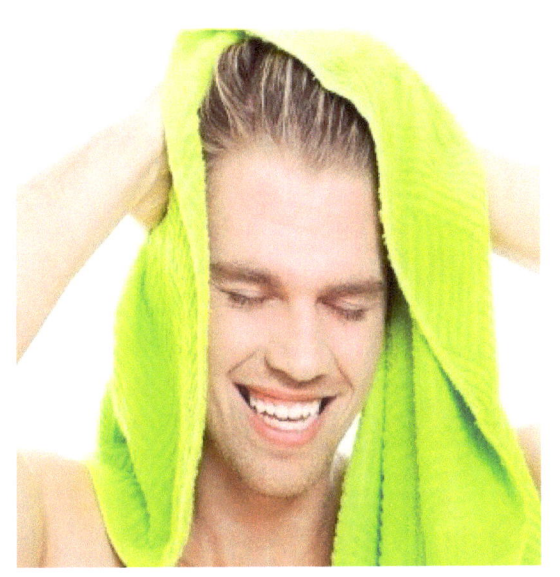

12

How to deal with wet hair

Be gentle with your hair when it's wet: hair has a tendency to fall easily when it's wet, so be gentle. When you shower be careful when you dry your hair, wet hair breaks easily. That's why you need to press gently the towel and let absorb the water: that's how one should dry its hair.

Wash your hair with cool water (not too hot) Hot water open your pores and could make your hair fall.

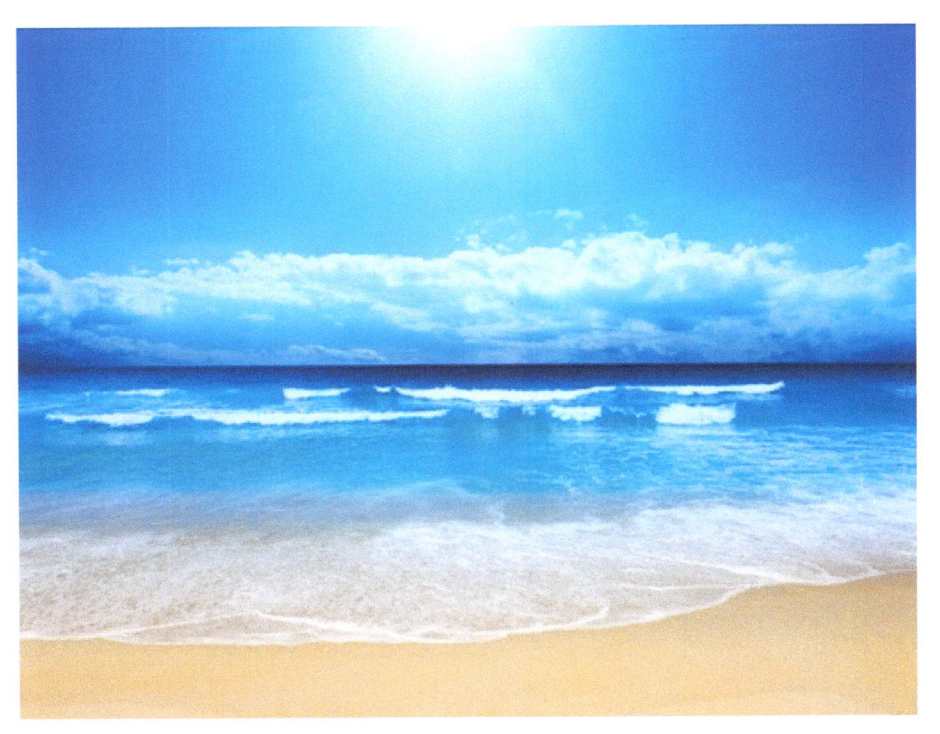

13

Go to the beach

Swimming in the beach (not the swimming pool) is good for your hair.
If you can find a natural lake it's good too.
Nature is good for your hair.

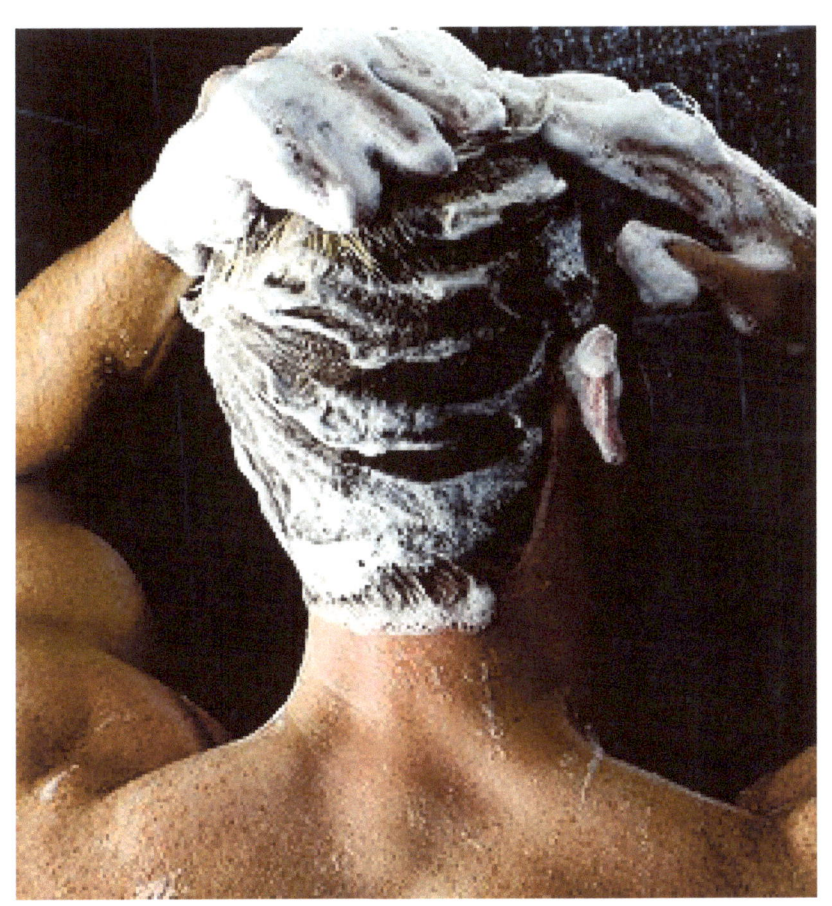

14

Wash your hair

Keep your hair clean: wash it at least 3 times a weeks. This will keep the pores of your scalp clean and open to prevent hair loss. Use good product: seek a good natural shampoo. A good quality shampoo is very important because it could stimulate your scalp and make your hair grow again. There are many good quality shampoos out there.

Have Faith

15

Be optimistic

Believe that this program will work and that you will stop and reverse hair loss: have faith! When you are ill and you try to heal being positive and optimistic is very important in order to achieve the results you want.

Here is what i advice you to do: each month work on four or five from the things listed above. This way in a few months you will have tried them all and you won't get lost.
For example : Start by cutting your hair ;eat good meals with cereals protein and vegetables ; chew your meals hard ; sleep a lot don't set the alarm ; exercise outdoor ; if you exercise indoor spent 20 to 30 min outside for fresh air (park) ; Ground yourself; fast from sex and meditate.
Or if you want you can work on all the steps at the same time like a program for 90 days .
After just a few days you will see that your hair loss has diminished tremendously, you also feel good. After two or three month you will end hair loss completely!